Diabetes
Log Book

Belongs to

Name: _____

Adress: _____

_____

Email: _____

Mobile Telephone: _____

Home Telephone: _____

Fax: _____

Diabetes Log Book

Date:						M	T	W	T	F	S	S

	Meal	Cal	Fat	Carbs	Total Sugar	Added Sugar	Protein	Fiber
BREAKFAST								
	Breakfast Totals							
	Blood Glucose Level	Befor:				Time:		
		After:				Time:		

		Cal	Fat	Carbs	Total Sugar	Added Sugar	Protein	Fiber
LUNCH								
	Lunch Totals							
	Blood Glucose Level	Befor:				Time:		
		After:				Time:		

		Cal	Fat	Carbs	Total Sugar	Added Sugar	Protein	Fiber
DINNER								
	Dinner Totals							
	Blood Glucose Level	Befor:				Time:		
		After:				Time:		

SNACKS								
	Snack Totals							

Daily Totals							

Bedtime Blood Glucose Level		Time:	

Water	Sleep	Medication	Activity	Minutes	Notes

Diabetes Log Book

Date:	M T W T F S S

	Meal	Cal	Fat	Carbs	Total Sugar	Added Sugar	Protein	Fiber
BREAKFAST								
	Breakfast Totals							
	Blood Glucose Level	Befor:				Time:		
		After:				Time:		

	Meal	Cal	Fat	Carbs	Total Sugar	Added Sugar	Protein	Fiber
LUNCH								
	Lunch Totals							
	Blood Glucose Level	Befor:				Time:		
		After:				Time:		

	Meal	Cal	Fat	Carbs	Total Sugar	Added Sugar	Protein	Fiber
DINNER								
	Dinner Totals							
	Blood Glucose Level	Befor:				Time:		
		After:				Time:		

SNACKS								
	Snack Totals							

Daily Totals							

Bedtime Blood Glucose Level		Time:	

Water	Sleep	Medication	Activity	Minutes	Notes

Diabetes Log Book

Date:						M	T	W	T	F	S	S

	Meal	Cal	Fat	Carbs	Total Sugar	Added Sugar	Protein	Fiber
BREAKFAST								
	Breakfast Totals							
	Blood Glucose Level	Befor:			Time:			
		After:			Time:			

		Cal	Fat	Carbs	Total Sugar	Added Sugar	Protein	Fiber
LUNCH								
	Lunch Totals							
	Blood Glucose Level	Befor:			Time:			
		After:			Time:			

		Cal	Fat	Carbs	Total Sugar	Added Sugar	Protein	Fiber
DINNER								
	DinnerTotals							
	Blood Glucose Level	Befor:			Time:			
		After:			Time:			

SNACKS								
	Snack Totals							

Daily Totals						

Bedtime Blood Glucose Level		Time:	

Water	Sleep	Medication	Activity	Minutes	Notes

Diabetes Log Book

| Date: | | | | | | M | T | W | T | F | S | S |

	Meal	Cal	Fat	Carbs	Total Sugar	Added Sugar	Protein	Fiber
BREAKFAST								
	Breakfast Totals							
	Blood Glucose Level	Befor:				Time:		
		After:				Time:		

LUNCH								
	Lunch Totals							
	Blood Glucose Level	Befor:				Time:		
		After:				Time:		

DINNER								
	DinnerTotals							
	Blood Glucose Level	Befor:				Time:		
		After:				Time:		

SNACKS								
	Snack Totals							

Daily Totals							

Bedtime Blood Glucose Level		Time:	

Water	Sleep	Medication	Activity	Minutes	Notes

Diabetes Log Book

Date:	M T W T F S S

	Meal	Cal	Fat	Carbs	Total Sugar	Added Sugar	Protein	Fiber
BREAKFAST								
	Breakfast Totals							
	Blood Glucose Level	Befor:			Time:			
		After:			Time:			

	Meal	Cal	Fat	Carbs	Total Sugar	Added Sugar	Protein	Fiber
LUNCH								
	Lunch Totals							
	Blood Glucose Level	Befor:			Time:			
		After:			Time:			

	Meal	Cal	Fat	Carbs	Total Sugar	Added Sugar	Protein	Fiber
DINNER								
	DinnerTotals							
	Blood Glucose Level	Befor:			Time:			
		After:			Time:			

	SNACKS							
	Snack Totals							

Daily Totals							

Bedtime Blood Glucose Level		Time:

Water	Sleep	Medication	Activity	Minutes	Notes

Notes

Diabetes Log Book

Date:					M T W T F S S			

	Meal	Cal	Fat	Carbs	Total Sugar	Added Sugar	Protein	Fiber
BREAKFAST								
	Breakfast Totals							
	Blood Glucose Level	Befor:			Time:			
		After:			Time:			
LUNCH								
	Lunch Totals							
	Blood Glucose Level	Befor:			Time:			
		After:			Time:			
DINNER								
	Dinner Totals							
	Blood Glucose Level	Befor:			Time:			
		After:			Time:			
SNACKS								
	Snack Totals							
	Daily Totals							

Bedtime Blood Glucose Level		Time:	

Water	Sleep	Medication	Activity	Minutes	Notes

Diabetes Log Book

Date:						M T W T F S S			

	Meal	Cal	Fat	Carbs	Total Sugar	Added Sugar	Protein	Fiber
BREAKFAST								
	Breakfast Totals							
	Blood Glucose Level	Befor:			Time:			
		After:			Time:			

	Meal	Cal	Fat	Carbs	Total Sugar	Added Sugar	Protein	Fiber
LUNCH								
	Lunch Totals							
	Blood Glucose Level	Befor:			Time:			
		After:			Time:			

	Meal	Cal	Fat	Carbs	Total Sugar	Added Sugar	Protein	Fiber
DINNER								
	Dinner Totals							
	Blood Glucose Level	Befor:			Time:			
		After:			Time:			

SNACKS								
	Snack Totals							

Daily Totals							

Bedtime Blood Glucose Level		Time:	

Water	Sleep	Medication	Activity	Minutes	Notes

Diabetes Log Book

Date:				M T W T F S S			

	Meal	Cal	Fat	Carbs	Total Sugar	Added Sugar	Protein	Fiber
BREAKFAST								
	Breakfast Totals							
	Blood Glucose Level	Befor:				Time:		
		After:				Time:		
LUNCH								
	Lunch Totals							
	Blood Glucose Level	Befor:				Time:		
		After:				Time:		
DINNER								
	Dinner Totals							
	Blood Glucose Level	Befor:				Time:		
		After:				Time:		
SNACKS								
	Snack Totals							

Daily Totals							

Bedtime Blood Glucose Level		Time:	

Water	Sleep	Medication	Activity	Minutes	Notes

Diabetes Log Book

Date:				M	T W	T	F	S S

	Meal	Cal	Fat	Carbs	Total Sugar	Added Sugar	Protein	Fiber
BREAKFAST								
	Breakfast Totals							
	Blood Glucose Level	Befor:				Time:		
		After:				Time:		

LUNCH								
	Lunch Totals							
	Blood Glucose Level	Befor:				Time:		
		After:				Time:		

DINNER								
	DinnerTotals							
	Blood Glucose Level	Befor:				Time:		
		After:				Time:		

SNACKS								
	Snack Totals							

Daily Totals							

Bedtime Blood Glucose Level		Time:	

Water	Sleep	Medication	Activity	Minutes	Notes

Diabetes Log Book

Date:					M	T	W	T	F	S	S

	Meal	Cal	Fat	Carbs	Total Sugar	Added Sugar	Protein	Fiber
BREAKFAST								
	Breakfast Totals							
	Blood Glucose Level	Befor:				Time:		
		After:				Time:		

	Meal							
LUNCH								
	Lunch Totals							
	Blood Glucose Level	Befor:				Time:		
		After:				Time:		

	Meal							
DINNER								
	Dinner Totals							
	Blood Glucose Level	Befor:				Time:		
		After:				Time:		

SNACKS								
	Snack Totals							

Daily Totals							

Bedtime Blood Glucose Level		Time:	

Water	Sleep	Medication	Activity	Minutes	Notes

Notes

Diabetes Log Book

Date:					M	T	W	T	F	S	S

	Meal	Cal	Fat	Carbs	Total Sugar	Added Sugar	Protein	Fiber
BREAKFAST								
	Breakfast Totals							
	Blood Glucose Level	Befor:			Time:			
		After:			Time:			

		Cal	Fat	Carbs	Total Sugar	Added Sugar	Protein	Fiber
LUNCH								
	Lunch Totals							
	Blood Glucose Level	Befor:			Time:			
		After:			Time:			

		Cal	Fat	Carbs	Total Sugar	Added Sugar	Protein	Fiber
DINNER								
	Dinner Totals							
	Blood Glucose Level	Befor:			Time:			
		After:			Time:			

SNACKS								
	Snack Totals							

Daily Totals							

Bedtime Blood Glucose Level		Time:	

Water	Sleep	Medication	Activity	Minutes	Notes

Diabetes Log Book

Date:								M T W T F S S		

	Meal	Cal	Fat	Carbs	Total Sugar	Added Sugar	Protein	Fiber
BREAKFAST								
	Breakfast Totals							
	Blood Glucose Level	Befor:				Time:		
		After:				Time:		

	Meal							
LUNCH								
	Lunch Totals							
	Blood Glucose Level	Befor:				Time:		
		After:				Time:		

	Meal							
DINNER								
	Dinner Totals							
	Blood Glucose Level	Befor:				Time:		
		After:				Time:		

SNACKS								
	Snack Totals							

Daily Totals							

Bedtime Blood Glucose Level		Time:	

Water	Sleep	Medication	Activity	Minutes	Notes

Diabetes Log Book

| Date: | | | | | M | T | W | T | F | S | S |

	Meal	Cal	Fat	Carbs	Total Sugar	Added Sugar	Protein	Fiber
BREAKFAST								
	Breakfast Totals							
	Blood Glucose Level	Befor:				Time:		
		After:				Time:		

	Meal	Cal	Fat	Carbs	Total Sugar	Added Sugar	Protein	Fiber
LUNCH								
	Lunch Totals							
	Blood Glucose Level	Befor:				Time:		
		After:				Time:		

	Meal	Cal	Fat	Carbs	Total Sugar	Added Sugar	Protein	Fiber
DINNER								
	Dinner Totals							
	Blood Glucose Level	Befor:				Time:		
		After:				Time:		

SNACKS								
	Snack Totals							

Daily Totals							

Bedtime Blood Glucose Level		Time:	

Water	Sleep	Medication	Activity	Minutes	Notes

Diabetes Log Book

| Date: | | | | | M T W T F S S | | | |

Meal		Cal	Fat	Carbs	Total Sugar	Added Sugar	Protein	Fiber
BREAKFAST								
	Breakfast Totals							
	Blood Glucose Level	Befor:				Time:		
		After:				Time:		

LUNCH								
	Lunch Totals							
	Blood Glucose Level	Befor:				Time:		
		After:				Time:		

DINNER								
	DinnerTotals							
	Blood Glucose Level	Befor:				Time:		
		After:				Time:		

SNACKS								
	Snack Totals							

Daily Totals							

Bedtime Blood Glucose Level		Time:	

Water	Sleep	Medication	Activity	Minutes	Notes

Diabetes Log Book

| Date: | | | | | | M T W T F S S | | | |

	Meal	Cal	Fat	Carbs	Total Sugar	Added Sugar	Protein	Fiber
BREAKFAST								
	Breakfast Totals							
	Blood Glucose Level	Befor:			Time:			
		After:			Time:			

LUNCH								
	Lunch Totals							
	Blood Glucose Level	Befor:			Time:			
		After:			Time:			

DINNER								
	Dinner Totals							
	Blood Glucose Level	Befor:			Time:			
		After:			Time:			

SNACKS								
	Snack Totals							

Daily Totals							

Bedtime Blood Glucose Level		Time:	

Water	Sleep	Medication	Activity	Minutes	Notes

Diabetes Log Book

| Date: | | | | | | M | T | W | T | F | S | S |

	Meal	Cal	Fat	Carbs	Total Sugar	Added Sugar	Protein	Fiber
BREAKFAST								
	Breakfast Totals							
	Blood Glucose Level	Befor:				Time:		
		After:				Time:		

		Cal	Fat	Carbs	Total Sugar	Added Sugar	Protein	Fiber
LUNCH								
	Lunch Totals							
	Blood Glucose Level	Befor:				Time:		
		After:				Time:		

		Cal	Fat	Carbs	Total Sugar	Added Sugar	Protein	Fiber
DINNER								
	Dinner Totals							
	Blood Glucose Level	Befor:				Time:		
		After:				Time:		

SNACKS								
	Snack Totals							

Daily Totals							

Bedtime Blood Glucose Level		Time:	

Water	Sleep	Medication	Activity	Minutes	Notes

Notes

Diabetes Log Book

Date:						M T W T F S S			

	Meal	Cal	Fat	Carbs	Total Sugar	Added Sugar	Protein	Fiber
BREAKFAST								
	Breakfast Totals							
	Blood Glucose Level	Befor:				Time:		
		After:				Time:		

LUNCH								
	Lunch Totals							
	Blood Glucose Level	Befor:				Time:		
		After:				Time:		

DINNER								
	Dinner Totals							
	Blood Glucose Level	Befor:				Time:		
		After:				Time:		

SNACKS								
	Snack Totals							

Daily Totals							

Bedtime Blood Glucose Level		Time:	

Water	Sleep	Medication	Activity	Minutes	Notes

Diabetes Log Book

Date:					M	T	W	T	F	S	S

	Meal	Cal	Fat	Carbs	Total Sugar	Added Sugar	Protein	Fiber
BREAKFAST								
	Breakfast Totals							
	Blood Glucose Level	Befor:				Time:		
		After:				Time:		

LUNCH								
	Lunch Totals							
	Blood Glucose Level	Befor:				Time:		
		After:				Time:		

DINNER								
	Dinner Totals							
	Blood Glucose Level	Befor:				Time:		
		After:				Time:		

SNACKS								
	Snack Totals							

Daily Totals						

Bedtime Blood Glucose Level		Time:	

Water	Sleep	Medication	Activity	Minutes	Notes

Diabetes Log Book

Date:						M T W T F S S			

	Meal	Cal	Fat	Carbs	Total Sugar	Added Sugar	Protein	Fiber
BREAKFAST								
	Breakfast Totals							
	Blood Glucose Level	Befor:				Time:		
		After:				Time:		

		Cal	Fat	Carbs	Total Sugar	Added Sugar	Protein	Fiber
LUNCH								
	Lunch Totals							
	Blood Glucose Level	Befor:				Time:		
		After:				Time:		

		Cal	Fat	Carbs	Total Sugar	Added Sugar	Protein	Fiber
DINNER								
	Dinner Totals							
	Blood Glucose Level	Befor:				Time:		
		After:				Time:		

SNACKS								
	Snack Totals							

Daily Totals							

Bedtime Blood Glucose Level		Time:	

Water	Sleep	Medication	Activity	Minutes	Notes

Diabetes Log Book

| Date: | | | | | M | T | W | T | F | S | S |

	Meal	Cal	Fat	Carbs	Total Sugar	Added Sugar	Protein	Fiber
BREAKFAST								
	Breakfast Totals							
	Blood Glucose Level	Befor:			Time:			
		After:			Time:			

		Cal	Fat	Carbs	Total Sugar	Added Sugar	Protein	Fiber
LUNCH								
	Lunch Totals							
	Blood Glucose Level	Befor:			Time:			
		After:			Time:			

		Cal	Fat	Carbs	Total Sugar	Added Sugar	Protein	Fiber
DINNER								
	Dinner Totals							
	Blood Glucose Level	Befor:			Time:			
		After:			Time:			

SNACKS								
	Snack Totals							

Daily Totals							

Bedtime Blood Glucose Level		Time:	

Water	Sleep	Medication	Activity	Minutes	Notes

Diabetes Log Book

| Date: | | | | | | M | T | W | T | F | S | S |

	Meal	Cal	Fat	Carbs	Total Sugar	Added Sugar	Protein	Fiber
BREAKFAST								
	Breakfast Totals							
	Blood Glucose Level	Befor:				Time:		
		After:				Time:		
LUNCH								
	Lunch Totals							
	Blood Glucose Level	Befor:				Time:		
		After:				Time:		
DINNER								
	Dinner Totals							
	Blood Glucose Level	Befor:				Time:		
		After:				Time:		
SNACKS								
	Snack Totals							

| | Daily Totals | | | | | | | |

| Bedtime Blood Glucose Level | | Time: |

Water	Sleep	Medication	Activity	Minutes	Notes

Notes

Diabetes Log Book

| Date: | | | | | | M T W T F S S | | | |

	Meal	Cal	Fat	Carbs	Total Sugar	Added Sugar	Protein	Fiber
BREAKFAST								
	Breakfast Totals							
	Blood Glucose Level	Befor:				Time:		
		After:				Time:		

	Meal	Cal	Fat	Carbs	Total Sugar	Added Sugar	Protein	Fiber
LUNCH								
	Lunch Totals							
	Blood Glucose Level	Befor:				Time:		
		After:				Time:		

	Meal	Cal	Fat	Carbs	Total Sugar	Added Sugar	Protein	Fiber
DINNER								
	Dinner Totals							
	Blood Glucose Level	Befor:				Time:		
		After:				Time:		

SNACKS								
	Snack Totals							

Daily Totals								

Bedtime Blood Glucose Level		Time:	

Water	Sleep	Medication	Activity	Minutes	Notes

Diabetes Log Book

Date:					M	T	W	T	F	S	S

	Meal	Cal	Fat	Carbs	Total Sugar	Added Sugar	Protein	Fiber
BREAKFAST								
	Breakfast Totals							
	Blood Glucose Level	Befor:				Time:		
		After:				Time:		

LUNCH								
	Lunch Totals							
	Blood Glucose Level	Befor:				Time:		
		After:				Time:		

DINNER								
	Dinner Totals							
	Blood Glucose Level	Befor:				Time:		
		After:				Time:		

SNACKS								
	Snack Totals							

Daily Totals							

Bedtime Blood Glucose Level		Time:	

Water	Sleep	Medication	Activity	Minutes	Notes

Diabetes Log Book

| Date: | | | | | M T W T F S S | | | |

	Meal	Cal	Fat	Carbs	Total Sugar	Added Sugar	Protein	Fiber
BREAKFAST								
	Breakfast Totals							
	Blood Glucose Level	Befor:				Time:		
		After:				Time:		

	Meal							
LUNCH								
	Lunch Totals							
	Blood Glucose Level	Befor:				Time:		
		After:				Time:		

	Meal							
DINNER								
	Dinner Totals							
	Blood Glucose Level	Befor:				Time:		
		After:				Time:		

SNACKS								
	Snack Totals							

Daily Totals							

Bedtime Blood Glucose Level		Time:	

Water	Sleep	Medication	Activity	Minutes	Notes

Diabetes Log Book

Date:				M T W T F S S			

	Meal	Cal	Fat	Carbs	Total Sugar	Added Sugar	Protein	Fiber
BREAKFAST								
	Breakfast Totals							
	Blood Glucose Level	Befor:			Time:			
		After:			Time:			

		Cal	Fat	Carbs	Total Sugar	Added Sugar	Protein	Fiber
LUNCH								
	Lunch Totals							
	Blood Glucose Level	Befor:			Time:			
		After:			Time:			

		Cal	Fat	Carbs	Total Sugar	Added Sugar	Protein	Fiber
DINNER								
	Dinner Totals							
	Blood Glucose Level	Befor:			Time:			
		After:			Time:			

SNACKS								
	Snack Totals							

Daily Totals							

Bedtime Blood Glucose Level		Time:	

Water	Sleep	Medication	Activity	Minutes	Notes

Diabetes Log Book

Date:							M T W T F S S		

	Meal	Cal	Fat	Carbs	Total Sugar	Added Sugar	Protein	Fiber
BREAKFAST								
	Breakfast Totals							
	Blood Glucose Level	Befor:				Time:		
		After:				Time:		

LUNCH								
	Lunch Totals							
	Blood Glucose Level	Befor:				Time:		
		After:				Time:		

DINNER								
	Dinner Totals							
	Blood Glucose Level	Befor:				Time:		
		After:				Time:		

SNACKS								
	Snack Totals							

	Daily Totals							

Bedtime Blood Glucose Level		Time:

Water	Sleep	Medication	Activity	Minutes	Notes

Diabetes Log Book

| Date: | | | | | M | T | W | T | F | S | S |

	Meal	Cal	Fat	Carbs	Total Sugar	Added Sugar	Protein	Fiber
BREAKFAST								
	Breakfast Totals							
	Blood Glucose Level	Befor:			Time:			
		After:			Time:			

		Cal	Fat	Carbs	Total Sugar	Added Sugar	Protein	Fiber
LUNCH								
	Lunch Totals							
	Blood Glucose Level	Befor:			Time:			
		After:			Time:			

		Cal	Fat	Carbs	Total Sugar	Added Sugar	Protein	Fiber
DINNER								
	Dinner Totals							
	Blood Glucose Level	Befor:			Time:			
		After:			Time:			

SNACKS								
	Snack Totals							

Daily Totals							

Bedtime Blood Glucose Level		Time:	

Water	Sleep	Medication	Activity	Minutes	Notes

Notes

Diabetes Log Book

Date:						M T W T F S S			

	Meal	Cal	Fat	Carbs	Total Sugar	Added Sugar	Protein	Fiber
BREAKFAST								
	Breakfast Totals							
	Blood Glucose Level	Befor:				Time:		
		After:				Time:		

LUNCH								
	Lunch Totals							
	Blood Glucose Level	Befor:				Time:		
		After:				Time:		

DINNER								
	DinnerTotals							
	Blood Glucose Level	Befor:				Time:		
		After:				Time:		

SNACKS								
	Snack Totals							

Daily Totals							

Bedtime Blood Glucose Level		Time:	

Water	Sleep	Medication	Activity	Minutes	Notes

Diabetes Log Book

| Date: | | | | | M T W T F S S | | | |

	Meal	Cal	Fat	Carbs	Total Sugar	Added Sugar	Protein	Fiber
BREAKFAST								
	Breakfast Totals							
	Blood Glucose Level	Befor:				Time:		
		After:				Time:		

LUNCH								
	Lunch Totals							
	Blood Glucose Level	Befor:				Time:		
		After:				Time:		

DINNER								
	Dinner Totals							
	Blood Glucose Level	Befor:				Time:		
		After:				Time:		

SNACKS								
	Snack Totals							

Daily Totals							

Bedtime Blood Glucose Level		Time:	

Water	Sleep	Medication	Activity	Minutes	Notes

Diabetes Log Book

Date:					M T W T F S S			

	Meal	Cal	Fat	Carbs	Total Sugar	Added Sugar	Protein	Fiber
BREAKFAST								
	Breakfast Totals							
	Blood Glucose Level	Befor:			Time:			
		After:			Time:			

	Meal	Cal	Fat	Carbs	Total Sugar	Added Sugar	Protein	Fiber
LUNCH								
	Lunch Totals							
	Blood Glucose Level	Befor:			Time:			
		After:			Time:			

	Meal	Cal	Fat	Carbs	Total Sugar	Added Sugar	Protein	Fiber
DINNER								
	Dinner Totals							
	Blood Glucose Level	Befor:			Time:			
		After:			Time:			

SNACKS								
	Snack Totals							

Daily Totals							

Bedtime Blood Glucose Level		Time:	

Water	Sleep	Medication	Activity	Minutes	Notes

Diabetes Log Book

Date:						M T W T F S S			

	Meal	Cal	Fat	Carbs	Total Sugar	Added Sugar	Protein	Fiber
BREAKFAST								
	Breakfast Totals							
	Blood Glucose Level	Befor:				Time:		
		After:				Time:		

LUNCH								
	Lunch Totals							
	Blood Glucose Level	Befor:				Time:		
		After:				Time:		

DINNER								
	Dinner Totals							
	Blood Glucose Level	Befor:				Time:		
		After:				Time:		

SNACKS								
	Snack Totals							

Daily Totals							

Bedtime Blood Glucose Level		Time:	

Water	Sleep	Medication	Activity	Minutes	Notes

Diabetes Log Book

| Date: | | | | M T W T F S S | | | |

	Meal	Cal	Fat	Carbs	Total Sugar	Added Sugar	Protein	Fiber
BREAKFAST								
	Breakfast Totals							
	Blood Glucose Level	Befor:			Time:			
		After:			Time:			

LUNCH								
	Lunch Totals							
	Blood Glucose Level	Befor:			Time:			
		After:			Time:			

DINNER								
	Dinner Totals							
	Blood Glucose Level	Befor:			Time:			
		After:			Time:			

SNACKS								
	Snack Totals							

Daily Totals							

Bedtime Blood Glucose Level		Time:	

Water	Sleep	Medication	Activity	Minutes	Notes

Notes

Diabetes Log Book

Date:					M	T	W	T	F	S	S

	Meal	Cal	Fat	Carbs	Total Sugar	Added Sugar	Protein	Fiber
BREAKFAST								
	Breakfast Totals							
	Blood Glucose Level	Befor:				Time:		
		After:				Time:		
LUNCH								
	Lunch Totals							
	Blood Glucose Level	Befor:				Time:		
		After:				Time:		
DINNER								
	Dinner Totals							
	Blood Glucose Level	Befor:				Time:		
		After:				Time:		
SNACKS								
	Snack Totals							

Daily Totals							

Bedtime Blood Glucose Level		Time:	

Water	Sleep	Medication	Activity	Minutes	Notes

Diabetes Log Book

Date:						M T W T F S S		

	Meal	Cal	Fat	Carbs	Total Sugar	Added Sugar	Protein	Fiber
BREAKFAST								
	Breakfast Totals							
	Blood Glucose Level	Befor:				Time:		
		After:				Time:		

		Cal	Fat	Carbs	Total Sugar	Added Sugar	Protein	Fiber
LUNCH								
	Lunch Totals							
	Blood Glucose Level	Befor:				Time:		
		After:				Time:		

		Cal	Fat	Carbs	Total Sugar	Added Sugar	Protein	Fiber
DINNER								
	DinnerTotals							
	Blood Glucose Level	Befor:				Time:		
		After:				Time:		

SNACKS								
	Snack Totals							

Daily Totals							

Bedtime Blood Glucose Level		Time:	

Water	Sleep	Medication	Activity	Minutes	Notes

Diabetes Log Book

| Date: | | | | | | M T W T F S S | | | |

	Meal	Cal	Fat	Carbs	Total Sugar	Added Sugar	Protein	Fiber
BREAKFAST								
	Breakfast Totals							
	Blood Glucose Level	Befor:			Time:			
		After:			Time:			

LUNCH								
	Lunch Totals							
	Blood Glucose Level	Befor:			Time:			
		After:			Time:			

DINNER								
	Dinner Totals							
	Blood Glucose Level	Befor:			Time:			
		After:			Time:			

SNACKS								
	Snack Totals							

Daily Totals						

Bedtime Blood Glucose Level		Time:	

Water	Sleep	Medication	Activity	Minutes	Notes

Diabetes Log Book

Date:						M T W T F S S			

	Meal	Cal	Fat	Carbs	Total Sugar	Added Sugar	Protein	Fiber
BREAKFAST								
	Breakfast Totals							
	Blood Glucose Level	Befor:				Time:		
		After:				Time:		

	Meal	Cal	Fat	Carbs	Total Sugar	Added Sugar	Protein	Fiber
LUNCH								
	Lunch Totals							
	Blood Glucose Level	Befor:				Time:		
		After:				Time:		

	Meal	Cal	Fat	Carbs	Total Sugar	Added Sugar	Protein	Fiber
DINNER								
	Dinner Totals							
	Blood Glucose Level	Befor:				Time:		
		After:				Time:		

SNACKS								
	Snack Totals							

Daily Totals							

Bedtime Blood Glucose Level		Time:	

Water	Sleep	Medication	Activity	Minutes	Notes

Diabetes Log Book

| Date: | | | | M T W T F S S | | | |

	Meal	Cal	Fat	Carbs	Total Sugar	Added Sugar	Protein	Fiber
BREAKFAST								
	Breakfast Totals							
	Blood Glucose Level	Befor:			Time:			
		After:			Time:			

LUNCH								
	Lunch Totals							
	Blood Glucose Level	Befor:			Time:			
		After:			Time:			

DINNER								
	Dinner Totals							
	Blood Glucose Level	Befor:			Time:			
		After:			Time:			

SNACKS								
	Snack Totals							

| Daily Totals | | | | | | | |

| Bedtime Blood Glucose Level | | Time: | |

Water	Sleep	Medication	Activity	Minutes	Notes

Notes

Diabetes Log Book

Date:					M T W T F S S			

	Meal	Cal	Fat	Carbs	Total Sugar	Added Sugar	Protein	Fiber
BREAKFAST								
	Breakfast Totals							
	Blood Glucose Level	Befor:				Time:		
		After:				Time:		
LUNCH								
	Lunch Totals							
	Blood Glucose Level	Befor:				Time:		
		After:				Time:		
DINNER								
	Dinner Totals							
	Blood Glucose Level	Befor:				Time:		
		After:				Time:		
SNACKS								
	Snack Totals							

	Daily Totals							

Bedtime Blood Glucose Level		Time:	

Water	Sleep	Medication	Activity	Minutes	Notes

Diabetes Log Book

| Date: | | | | M | T | W | T | F | S | S |

	Meal	Cal	Fat	Carbs	Total Sugar	Added Sugar	Protein	Fiber
BREAKFAST								
	Breakfast Totals							
	Blood Glucose Level	Befor:				Time:		
		After:				Time:		

	Meal	Cal	Fat	Carbs	Total Sugar	Added Sugar	Protein	Fiber
LUNCH								
	Lunch Totals							
	Blood Glucose Level	Befor:				Time:		
		After:				Time:		

	Meal	Cal	Fat	Carbs	Total Sugar	Added Sugar	Protein	Fiber
DINNER								
	DinnerTotals							
	Blood Glucose Level	Befor:				Time:		
		After:				Time:		

SNACKS								
	Snack Totals							

Daily Totals							

Bedtime Blood Glucose Level		Time:	

Water	Sleep	Medication	Activity	Minutes	Notes

Diabetes Log Book

Date:						M T W T F S S			

	Meal	Cal	Fat	Carbs	Total Sugar	Added Sugar	Protein	Fiber
BREAKFAST								
	Breakfast Totals							
	Blood Glucose Level	Befor:				Time:		
		After:				Time:		

LUNCH								
	Lunch Totals							
	Blood Glucose Level	Befor:				Time:		
		After:				Time:		

DINNER								
	Dinner Totals							
	Blood Glucose Level	Befor:				Time:		
		After:				Time:		

SNACKS								
	Snack Totals							

Daily Totals							

Bedtime Blood Glucose Level		Time:	

Water	Sleep	Medication	Activity	Minutes	Notes

Diabetes Log Book

Date:						M T W T F S S			

	Meal	Cal	Fat	Carbs	Total Sugar	Added Sugar	Protein	Fiber
BREAKFAST								
	Breakfast Totals							
	Blood Glucose Level	Befor:				Time:		
		After:				Time:		

LUNCH								
	Lunch Totals							
	Blood Glucose Level	Befor:				Time:		
		After:				Time:		

DINNER								
	Dinner Totals							
	Blood Glucose Level	Befor:				Time:		
		After:				Time:		

SNACKS								
	Snack Totals							

Daily Totals							

Bedtime Blood Glucose Level		Time:	

Water	Sleep	Medication	Activity	Minutes	Notes

Diabetes Log Book

Date:					M T W T F S S			

	Meal	Cal	Fat	Carbs	Total Sugar	Added Sugar	Protein	Fiber
BREAKFAST								
	Breakfast Totals							
	Blood Glucose Level	Befor:				Time:		
		After:				Time:		

	Meal	Cal	Fat	Carbs	Total Sugar	Added Sugar	Protein	Fiber
LUNCH								
	Lunch Totals							
	Blood Glucose Level	Befor:				Time:		
		After:				Time:		

	Meal	Cal	Fat	Carbs	Total Sugar	Added Sugar	Protein	Fiber
DINNER								
	DinnerTotals							
	Blood Glucose Level	Befor:				Time:		
		After:				Time:		

SNACKS								
	Snack Totals							

Daily Totals							

Bedtime Blood Glucose Level		Time:	

Water	Sleep	Medication	Activity	Minutes	Notes

Notes

Diabetes Log Book

Date:					M	T	W	T	F	S	S

	Meal	Cal	Fat	Carbs	Total Sugar	Added Sugar	Protein	Fiber
BREAKFAST								
	Breakfast Totals							
	Blood Glucose Level	Befor: Time:						
		After: Time:						

		Cal	Fat	Carbs	Total Sugar	Added Sugar	Protein	Fiber
LUNCH								
	Lunch Totals							
	Blood Glucose Level	Befor: Time:						
		After: Time:						

		Cal	Fat	Carbs	Total Sugar	Added Sugar	Protein	Fiber
DINNER								
	Dinner Totals							
	Blood Glucose Level	Befor: Time:						
		After: Time:						

SNACKS								
	Snack Totals							

Daily Totals							

Bedtime Blood Glucose Level		Time:

Water	Sleep	Medication	Activity	Minutes	Notes

Diabetes Log Book

Date:						M T W T F S S			

	Meal	Cal	Fat	Carbs	Total Sugar	Added Sugar	Protein	Fiber
BREAKFAST								
	Breakfast Totals							
	Blood Glucose Level	Befor:				Time:		
		After:				Time:		

		Cal	Fat	Carbs	Total Sugar	Added Sugar	Protein	Fiber
LUNCH								
	Lunch Totals							
	Blood Glucose Level	Befor:				Time:		
		After:				Time:		

		Cal	Fat	Carbs	Total Sugar	Added Sugar	Protein	Fiber
DINNER								
	Dinner Totals							
	Blood Glucose Level	Befor:				Time:		
		After:				Time:		

SNACKS								
	Snack Totals							

Daily Totals								

Bedtime Blood Glucose Level		Time:	

Water	Sleep	Medication	Activity	Minutes	Notes

Diabetes Log Book

| Date: | | | | | M T W T F S S | | | |

	Meal	Cal	Fat	Carbs	Total Sugar	Added Sugar	Protein	Fiber
BREAKFAST								
	Breakfast Totals							
	Blood Glucose Level	Befor:			Time:			
		After:			Time:			

LUNCH								
	Lunch Totals							
	Blood Glucose Level	Befor:			Time:			
		After:			Time:			

DINNER								
	Dinner Totals							
	Blood Glucose Level	Befor:			Time:			
		After:			Time:			

SNACKS								
	Snack Totals							

Daily Totals							

Bedtime Blood Glucose Level		Time:	

Water	Sleep	Medication	Activity	Minutes	Notes

Diabetes Log Book

| Date: | | | | | | M | T | W | T | F | S | S |

	Meal	Cal	Fat	Carbs	Total Sugar	Added Sugar	Protein	Fiber
BREAKFAST								
	Breakfast Totals							
	Blood Glucose Level	Befor:				Time:		
		After:				Time:		

		Cal	Fat	Carbs	Total Sugar	Added Sugar	Protein	Fiber
LUNCH								
	Lunch Totals							
	Blood Glucose Level	Befor:				Time:		
		After:				Time:		

		Cal	Fat	Carbs	Total Sugar	Added Sugar	Protein	Fiber
DINNER								
	Dinner Totals							
	Blood Glucose Level	Befor:				Time:		
		After:				Time:		

SNACKS								
	Snack Totals							

Daily Totals							

Bedtime Blood Glucose Level		Time:	

Water	Sleep	Medication	Activity	Minutes	Notes

Diabetes Log Book

| Date: | | | | M T W T F S S | | | |

	Meal	Cal	Fat	Carbs	Total Sugar	Added Sugar	Protein	Fiber
BREAKFAST								
	Breakfast Totals							
	Blood Glucose Level	Befor:			Time:			
		After:			Time:			

	Meal							
LUNCH								
	Lunch Totals							
	Blood Glucose Level	Befor:			Time:			
		After:			Time:			

	Meal							
DINNER								
	Dinner Totals							
	Blood Glucose Level	Befor:			Time:			
		After:			Time:			

SNACKS								
	Snack Totals							

Daily Totals						

Bedtime Blood Glucose Level		Time:	

Water	Sleep	Medication	Activity	Minutes	Notes

Notes

Diabetes Log Book

Date:					M	T	W	T	F	S	S

	Meal	Cal	Fat	Carbs	Total Sugar	Added Sugar	Protein	Fiber
BREAKFAST								
	Breakfast Totals							
	Blood Glucose Level	Befor:				Time:		
		After:				Time:		

		Cal	Fat	Carbs	Total Sugar	Added Sugar	Protein	Fiber
LUNCH								
	Lunch Totals							
	Blood Glucose Level	Befor:				Time:		
		After:				Time:		

		Cal	Fat	Carbs	Total Sugar	Added Sugar	Protein	Fiber
DINNER								
	Dinner Totals							
	Blood Glucose Level	Befor:				Time:		
		After:				Time:		

SNACKS								
	Snack Totals							

Daily Totals						

Bedtime Blood Glucose Level		Time:	

Water	Sleep	Medication	Activity	Minutes	Notes

Diabetes Log Book

| Date: | | | | | | M T W T F S S | | | |

	Meal	Cal	Fat	Carbs	Total Sugar	Added Sugar	Protein	Fiber
BREAKFAST								
	Breakfast Totals							
	Blood Glucose Level	Befor:				Time:		
		After:				Time:		

	Meal	Cal	Fat	Carbs	Total Sugar	Added Sugar	Protein	Fiber
LUNCH								
	Lunch Totals							
	Blood Glucose Level	Befor:				Time:		
		After:				Time:		

	Meal	Cal	Fat	Carbs	Total Sugar	Added Sugar	Protein	Fiber
DINNER								
	Dinner Totals							
	Blood Glucose Level	Befor:				Time:		
		After:				Time:		

SNACKS								
	Snack Totals							

Daily Totals							

Bedtime Blood Glucose Level		Time:	

Water	Sleep	Medication	Activity	Minutes	Notes

Diabetes Log Book

Date:						M T W T F S S			

	Meal	Cal	Fat	Carbs	Total Sugar	Added Sugar	Protein	Fiber
BREAKFAST								
	Breakfast Totals							
	Blood Glucose Level	Befor:			Time:			
		After:			Time:			

LUNCH								
	Lunch Totals							
	Blood Glucose Level	Befor:			Time:			
		After:			Time:			

DINNER								
	Dinner Totals							
	Blood Glucose Level	Befor:			Time:			
		After:			Time:			

SNACKS								
	Snack Totals							

Daily Totals							

Bedtime Blood Glucose Level		Time:	

Water	Sleep	Medication	Activity	Minutes	Notes

Diabetes Log Book

Date:					M T W T F S S			

	Meal	Cal	Fat	Carbs	Total Sugar	Added Sugar	Protein	Fiber
BREAKFAST								
	Breakfast Totals							
	Blood Glucose Level	Befor:				Time:		
		After:				Time:		

LUNCH								
	Lunch Totals							
	Blood Glucose Level	Befor:				Time:		
		After:				Time:		

DINNER								
	Dinner Totals							
	Blood Glucose Level	Befor:				Time:		
		After:				Time:		

SNACKS								
	Snack Totals							

Daily Totals							

Bedtime Blood Glucose Level		Time:	

Water	Sleep	Medication	Activity	Minutes	Notes

Diabetes Log Book

Date:					M	T	W	T	F	S	S

	Meal	Cal	Fat	Carbs	Total Sugar	Added Sugar	Protein	Fiber
BREAKFAST								
	Breakfast Totals							
	Blood Glucose Level	Befor:				Time:		
		After:				Time:		

	Meal	Cal	Fat	Carbs	Total Sugar	Added Sugar	Protein	Fiber
LUNCH								
	Lunch Totals							
	Blood Glucose Level	Befor:				Time:		
		After:				Time:		

	Meal	Cal	Fat	Carbs	Total Sugar	Added Sugar	Protein	Fiber
DINNER								
	Dinner Totals							
	Blood Glucose Level	Befor:				Time:		
		After:				Time:		

		Cal	Fat	Carbs	Total Sugar	Added Sugar	Protein	Fiber
SNACKS								
	Snack Totals							

Daily Totals							

Bedtime Blood Glucose Level		Time:

Water	Sleep	Medication	Activity	Minutes	Notes

Notes

Diabetes Log Book

| Date: | | | | | M | T | W | T | F | S | S |

	Meal	Cal	Fat	Carbs	Total Sugar	Added Sugar	Protein	Fiber
BREAKFAST								
	Breakfast Totals							
	Blood Glucose Level	Befor:				Time:		
		After:				Time:		

		Cal	Fat	Carbs	Total Sugar	Added Sugar	Protein	Fiber
LUNCH								
	Lunch Totals							
	Blood Glucose Level	Befor:				Time:		
		After:				Time:		

		Cal	Fat	Carbs	Total Sugar	Added Sugar	Protein	Fiber
DINNER								
	DinnerTotals							
	Blood Glucose Level	Befor:				Time:		
		After:				Time:		

SNACKS								
	Snack Totals							

Daily Totals							

Bedtime Blood Glucose Level		Time:	

Water	Sleep	Medication	Activity	Minutes	Notes

Diabetes Log Book

Date:						M T W T F S S			

	Meal	Cal	Fat	Carbs	Total Sugar	Added Sugar	Protein	Fiber
BREAKFAST								
	Breakfast Totals							
	Blood Glucose Level	Befor:				Time:		
		After:				Time:		
LUNCH								
	Lunch Totals							
	Blood Glucose Level	Befor:				Time:		
		After:				Time:		
DINNER								
	Dinner Totals							
	Blood Glucose Level	Befor:				Time:		
		After:				Time:		
SNACKS								
	Snack Totals							

Daily Totals							

Bedtime Blood Glucose Level		Time:	

Water	Sleep	Medication	Activity	Minutes	Notes

Diabetes Log Book

Date:					M	T	W	T	F	S	S

	Meal	Cal	Fat	Carbs	Total Sugar	Added Sugar	Protein	Fiber
BREAKFAST								
	Breakfast Totals							
	Blood Glucose Level	Befor:			Time:			
		After:			Time:			

		Cal	Fat	Carbs	Total Sugar	Added Sugar	Protein	Fiber
LUNCH								
	Lunch Totals							
	Blood Glucose Level	Befor:			Time:			
		After:			Time:			

		Cal	Fat	Carbs	Total Sugar	Added Sugar	Protein	Fiber
DINNER								
	Dinner Totals							
	Blood Glucose Level	Befor:			Time:			
		After:			Time:			

SNACKS								
	Snack Totals							

Daily Totals							

Bedtime Blood Glucose Level		Time:	

Water	Sleep	Medication	Activity	Minutes	Notes

Diabetes Log Book

Date:					M T W T F S S			

	Meal	Cal	Fat	Carbs	Total Sugar	Added Sugar	Protein	Fiber
BREAKFAST								
	Breakfast Totals							
	Blood Glucose Level	Befor:				Time:		
		After:				Time:		

LUNCH								
	Lunch Totals							
	Blood Glucose Level	Befor:				Time:		
		After:				Time:		

DINNER								
	Dinner Totals							
	Blood Glucose Level	Befor:				Time:		
		After:				Time:		

SNACKS								
	Snack Totals							

Daily Totals							

Bedtime Blood Glucose Level		Time:	

Water	Sleep	Medication	Activity	Minutes	Notes

Diabetes Log Book

| Date: | | | | | M | T | W | T | F | S | S |

	Meal	Cal	Fat	Carbs	Total Sugar	Added Sugar	Protein	Fiber
BREAKFAST								
	Breakfast Totals							
	Blood Glucose Level	Befor:				Time:		
		After:				Time:		

	Meal	Cal	Fat	Carbs	Total Sugar	Added Sugar	Protein	Fiber
LUNCH								
	Lunch Totals							
	Blood Glucose Level	Befor:				Time:		
		After:				Time:		

	Meal	Cal	Fat	Carbs	Total Sugar	Added Sugar	Protein	Fiber
DINNER								
	Dinner Totals							
	Blood Glucose Level	Befor:				Time:		
		After:				Time:		

		Cal	Fat	Carbs	Total Sugar	Added Sugar	Protein	Fiber
SNACKS								
	Snack Totals							

| Daily Totals | | | | | | | |

| Bedtime Blood Glucose Level | | Time: | |

Water	Sleep	Medication	Activity	Minutes	Notes

Notes

Diabetes Log Book

Date:						M T W T F S S

BREAKFAST

Meal	Cal	Fat	Carbs	Total Sugar	Added Sugar	Protein	Fiber
Breakfast Totals							
Blood Glucose Level	Befor:			Time:			
	After:			Time:			

LUNCH

Meal	Cal	Fat	Carbs	Total Sugar	Added Sugar	Protein	Fiber
Lunch Totals							
Blood Glucose Level	Befor:			Time:			
	After:			Time:			

DINNER

Meal	Cal	Fat	Carbs	Total Sugar	Added Sugar	Protein	Fiber
Dinner Totals							
Blood Glucose Level	Befor:			Time:			
	After:			Time:			

SNACKS

Snack Totals							

Daily Totals							

Bedtime Blood Glucose Level		Time:	

Water	Sleep	Medication	Activity	Minutes	Notes

Diabetes Log Book

Date:						M	T	W	T	F	S	S

	Meal	Cal	Fat	Carbs	Total Sugar	Added Sugar	Protein	Fiber
BREAKFAST								
	Breakfast Totals							
	Blood Glucose Level	Befor:				Time:		
		After:				Time:		

		Cal	Fat	Carbs	Total Sugar	Added Sugar	Protein	Fiber
LUNCH								
	Lunch Totals							
	Blood Glucose Level	Befor:				Time:		
		After:				Time:		

		Cal	Fat	Carbs	Total Sugar	Added Sugar	Protein	Fiber
DINNER								
	Dinner Totals							
	Blood Glucose Level	Befor:				Time:		
		After:				Time:		

SNACKS								
	Snack Totals							

Daily Totals							

Bedtime Blood Glucose Level		Time:	

Water	Sleep	Medication	Activity	Minutes	Notes

Diabetes Log Book

| Date: | | | | | | M T W T F S S | | | |

	Meal	Cal	Fat	Carbs	Total Sugar	Added Sugar	Protein	Fiber
BREAKFAST								
	Breakfast Totals							
	Blood Glucose Level	Befor:			Time:			
		After:			Time:			

LUNCH								
	Lunch Totals							
	Blood Glucose Level	Befor:			Time:			
		After:			Time:			

DINNER								
	Dinner Totals							
	Blood Glucose Level	Befor:			Time:			
		After:			Time:			

SNACKS								
	Snack Totals							

Daily Totals							

Bedtime Blood Glucose Level		Time:	

Water	Sleep	Medication	Activity	Minutes	Notes

Diabetes Log Book

Date:							M T W T F S S		

	Meal	Cal	Fat	Carbs	Total Sugar	Added Sugar	Protein	Fiber
BREAKFAST								
	Breakfast Totals							
	Blood Glucose Level	Befor:			Time:			
		After:			Time:			

LUNCH								
	Lunch Totals							
	Blood Glucose Level	Befor:			Time:			
		After:			Time:			

DINNER								
	Dinner Totals							
	Blood Glucose Level	Befor:			Time:			
		After:			Time:			

SNACKS								
	Snack Totals							

Daily Totals							

Bedtime Blood Glucose Level		Time:	

Water	Sleep	Medication	Activity	Minutes	Notes

Diabetes Log Book

Date:					M	T	W	T	F	S	S

	Meal	Cal	Fat	Carbs	Total Sugar	Added Sugar	Protein	Fiber
BREAKFAST								
	Breakfast Totals							
	Blood Glucose Level	Befor:				Time:		
		After:				Time:		
LUNCH								
	Lunch Totals							
	Blood Glucose Level	Befor:				Time:		
		After:				Time:		
DINNER								
	Dinner Totals							
	Blood Glucose Level	Befor:				Time:		
		After:				Time:		
SNACKS								
	Snack Totals							
	Daily Totals							

Bedtime Blood Glucose Level		Time:	

Water	Sleep	Medication	Activity	Minutes	Notes

Diabetes Log Book

Date:						M T W T F S S		

	Meal	Cal	Fat	Carbs	Total Sugar	Added Sugar	Protein	Fiber
BREAKFAST								
	Breakfast Totals							
	Blood Glucose Level	Befor:				Time:		
		After:				Time:		

LUNCH								
	Lunch Totals							
	Blood Glucose Level	Befor:				Time:		
		After:				Time:		

DINNER								
	Dinner Totals							
	Blood Glucose Level	Befor:				Time:		
		After:				Time:		

SNACKS								
	Snack Totals							

Daily Totals							

Bedtime Blood Glucose Level		Time:	

Water	Sleep	Medication	Activity	Minutes	Notes

Notes

Diabetes Log Book

| Date: | | | | | | M T W T F S S | | | |

	Meal	Cal	Fat	Carbs	Total Sugar	Added Sugar	Protein	Fiber
BREAKFAST								
	Breakfast Totals							
	Blood Glucose Level	Befor:				Time:		
		After:				Time:		

LUNCH								
	Lunch Totals							
	Blood Glucose Level	Befor:				Time:		
		After:				Time:		

DINNER								
	Dinner Totals							
	Blood Glucose Level	Befor:				Time:		
		After:				Time:		

SNACKS								
	Snack Totals							

Daily Totals							

Bedtime Blood Glucose Level		Time:	

Water	Sleep	Medication	Activity	Minutes	Notes

Diabetes Log Book

Date:				M T W T F S S			

	Meal	Cal	Fat	Carbs	Total Sugar	Added Sugar	Protein	Fiber
BREAKFAST								
	Breakfast Totals							
	Blood Glucose Level	Befor:				Time:		
		After:				Time:		

LUNCH								
	Lunch Totals							
	Blood Glucose Level	Befor:				Time:		
		After:				Time:		

DINNER								
	Dinner Totals							
	Blood Glucose Level	Befor:				Time:		
		After:				Time:		

SNACKS								
	Snack Totals							

Daily Totals							

Bedtime Blood Glucose Level		Time:	

Water	Sleep	Medication	Activity	Minutes	Notes

Diabetes Log Book

Date:							M	T	W	T	F	S	S

	Meal	Cal	Fat	Carbs	Total Sugar	Added Sugar	Protein	Fiber
BREAKFAST								
	Breakfast Totals							
	Blood Glucose Level	Befor:				Time:		
		After:				Time:		
LUNCH								
	Lunch Totals							
	Blood Glucose Level	Befor:				Time:		
		After:				Time:		
DINNER								
	Dinner Totals							
	Blood Glucose Level	Befor:				Time:		
		After:				Time:		
SNACKS								
	Snack Totals							
	Daily Totals							

Bedtime Blood Glucose Level		Time:	

Water	Sleep	Medication	Activity	Minutes	Notes

Diabetes Log Book

Date:					M	T	W	T	F	S	S

	Meal	Cal	Fat	Carbs	Total Sugar	Added Sugar	Protein	Fiber
BREAKFAST								
	Breakfast Totals							
	Blood Glucose Level	Befor:				Time:		
		After:				Time:		
LUNCH								
	Lunch Totals							
	Blood Glucose Level	Befor:				Time:		
		After:				Time:		
DINNER								
	Dinner Totals							
	Blood Glucose Level	Befor:				Time:		
		After:				Time:		
SNACKS								
	Snack Totals							
	Daily Totals							

Bedtime Blood Glucose Level		Time:

Water	Sleep	Medication	Activity	Minutes	Notes

Diabetes Log Book

| Date: | | | | | M | T | W | T | F | S | S |

	Meal	Cal	Fat	Carbs	Total Sugar	Added Sugar	Protein	Fiber
BREAKFAST								
	Breakfast Totals							
	Blood Glucose Level	Befor:				Time:		
		After:				Time:		

	Meal	Cal	Fat	Carbs	Total Sugar	Added Sugar	Protein	Fiber
LUNCH								
	Lunch Totals							
	Blood Glucose Level	Befor:				Time:		
		After:				Time:		

	Meal	Cal	Fat	Carbs	Total Sugar	Added Sugar	Protein	Fiber
DINNER								
	Dinner Totals							
	Blood Glucose Level	Befor:				Time:		
		After:				Time:		

SNACKS								
	Snack Totals							

Daily Totals							

Bedtime Blood Glucose Level		Time:	

Water	Sleep	Medication	Activity	Minutes	Notes

Notes

Diabetes Log Book

| Date: | | | | | M | T | W | T | F | S | S |

	Meal	Cal	Fat	Carbs	Total Sugar	Added Sugar	Protein	Fiber
BREAKFAST								
	Breakfast Totals							
	Blood Glucose Level	Befor:				Time:		
		After:				Time:		

	Meal	Cal	Fat	Carbs	Total Sugar	Added Sugar	Protein	Fiber
LUNCH								
	Lunch Totals							
	Blood Glucose Level	Befor:				Time:		
		After:				Time:		

	Meal	Cal	Fat	Carbs	Total Sugar	Added Sugar	Protein	Fiber
DINNER								
	DinnerTotals							
	Blood Glucose Level	Befor:				Time:		
		After:				Time:		

SNACKS								
	Snack Totals							

| Daily Totals | | | | | | | |

| Bedtime Blood Glucose Level | | | Time: | |

Water	Sleep	Medication	Activity	Minutes	Notes

Diabetes Log Book

| Date: | | | | | M T W T F S S | | | |

	Meal	Cal	Fat	Carbs	Total Sugar	Added Sugar	Protein	Fiber
BREAKFAST								
	Breakfast Totals							
	Blood Glucose Level	Befor:				Time:		
		After:				Time:		
LUNCH								
	Lunch Totals							
	Blood Glucose Level	Befor:				Time:		
		After:				Time:		
DINNER								
	Dinner Totals							
	Blood Glucose Level	Befor:				Time:		
		After:				Time:		
SNACKS								
	Snack Totals							
	Daily Totals							

| Bedtime Blood Glucose Level | | Time: | |

Water	Sleep	Medication	Activity	Minutes	Notes

Diabetes Log Book

Date:						M T W T F S S			

	Meal	Cal	Fat	Carbs	Total Sugar	Added Sugar	Protein	Fiber
BREAKFAST								
	Breakfast Totals							
	Blood Glucose Level	Befor:				Time:		
		After:				Time:		

LUNCH								
	Lunch Totals							
	Blood Glucose Level	Befor:				Time:		
		After:				Time:		

DINNER								
	Dinner Totals							
	Blood Glucose Level	Befor:				Time:		
		After:				Time:		

SNACKS								
	Snack Totals							

Daily Totals							

Bedtime Blood Glucose Level		Time:	

Water	Sleep	Medication	Activity	Minutes	Notes

Diabetes Log Book

Date:					M	T	W	T	F	S	S

	Meal	Cal	Fat	Carbs	Total Sugar	Added Sugar	Protein	Fiber
BREAKFAST								
	Breakfast Totals							
	Blood Glucose Level	Befor:				Time:		
		After:				Time:		

	Meal	Cal	Fat	Carbs	Total Sugar	Added Sugar	Protein	Fiber
LUNCH								
	Lunch Totals							
	Blood Glucose Level	Befor:				Time:		
		After:				Time:		

	Meal	Cal	Fat	Carbs	Total Sugar	Added Sugar	Protein	Fiber
DINNER								
	Dinner Totals							
	Blood Glucose Level	Befor:				Time:		
		After:				Time:		

		Cal	Fat	Carbs	Total Sugar	Added Sugar	Protein	Fiber
SNACKS								
	Snack Totals							

Daily Totals							

Bedtime Blood Glucose Level		Time:	

Water	Sleep	Medication	Activity	Minutes	Notes

Notes

Diabetes Log Book

Date:					M T W T F S S			

	Meal	Cal	Fat	Carbs	Total Sugar	Added Sugar	Protein	Fiber
BREAKFAST								
	Breakfast Totals							
	Blood Glucose Level	Befor:			Time:			
		After:			Time:			

LUNCH								
	Lunch Totals							
	Blood Glucose Level	Befor:			Time:			
		After:			Time:			

DINNER								
	Dinner Totals							
	Blood Glucose Level	Befor:			Time:			
		After:			Time:			

SNACKS								
	Snack Totals							

Daily Totals							

Bedtime Blood Glucose Level		Time:	

Water	Sleep	Medication	Activity	Minutes	Notes

Diabetes Log Book

Date:						M	T	W	T	F	S	S

	Meal	Cal	Fat	Carbs	Total Sugar	Added Sugar	Protein	Fiber
BREAKFAST								
	Breakfast Totals							
	Blood Glucose Level	Befor:				Time:		
		After:				Time:		

		Cal	Fat	Carbs	Total Sugar	Added Sugar	Protein	Fiber
LUNCH								
	Lunch Totals							
	Blood Glucose Level	Befor:				Time:		
		After:				Time:		

		Cal	Fat	Carbs	Total Sugar	Added Sugar	Protein	Fiber
DINNER								
	DinnerTotals							
	Blood Glucose Level	Befor:				Time:		
		After:				Time:		

SNACKS								
	Snack Totals							

Daily Totals							

Bedtime Blood Glucose Level		Time:	

Water	Sleep	Medication	Activity	Minutes	Notes

Diabetes Log Book

Date:					M T W T F S S			

	Meal	Cal	Fat	Carbs	Total Sugar	Added Sugar	Protein	Fiber
BREAKFAST								
	Breakfast Totals							
	Blood Glucose Level	Befor:				Time:		
		After:				Time:		

LUNCH								
	Lunch Totals							
	Blood Glucose Level	Befor:				Time:		
		After:				Time:		

DINNER								
	Dinner Totals							
	Blood Glucose Level	Befor:				Time:		
		After:				Time:		

SNACKS								
	Snack Totals							

Daily Totals							

Bedtime Blood Glucose Level		Time:	

Water	Sleep	Medication	Activity	Minutes	Notes

Diabetes Log Book

Date:				M T W T F S S			

	Meal	Cal	Fat	Carbs	Total Sugar	Added Sugar	Protein	Fiber
BREAKFAST								
	Breakfast Totals							
	Blood Glucose Level	Befor:				Time:		
		After:				Time:		

LUNCH								
	Lunch Totals							
	Blood Glucose Level	Befor:				Time:		
		After:				Time:		

DINNER								
	Dinner Totals							
	Blood Glucose Level	Befor:				Time:		
		After:				Time:		

SNACKS								
	Snack Totals							

Daily Totals							

Bedtime Blood Glucose Level		Time:	

Water	Sleep	Medication	Activity	Minutes	Notes

Diabetes Log Book

Date:					M	T	W	T	F	S	S

	Meal	Cal	Fat	Carbs	Total Sugar	Added Sugar	Protein	Fiber
BREAKFAST								
	Breakfast Totals							
	Blood Glucose Level	Befor:				Time:		
		After:				Time:		

		Cal	Fat	Carbs	Total Sugar	Added Sugar	Protein	Fiber
LUNCH								
	Lunch Totals							
	Blood Glucose Level	Befor:				Time:		
		After:				Time:		

		Cal	Fat	Carbs	Total Sugar	Added Sugar	Protein	Fiber
DINNER								
	Dinner Totals							
	Blood Glucose Level	Befor:				Time:		
		After:				Time:		

SNACKS								
	Snack Totals							

Daily Totals							

Bedtime Blood Glucose Level		Time:	

Water	Sleep	Medication	Activity	Minutes	Notes

Diabetes Log Book

Date:						M	T	W	T	F	S	S

	Meal	Cal	Fat	Carbs	Total Sugar	Added Sugar	Protein	Fiber
BREAKFAST								
	Breakfast Totals							
	Blood Glucose Level	Befor:				Time:		
		After:				Time:		

LUNCH								
	Lunch Totals							
	Blood Glucose Level	Befor:				Time:		
		After:				Time:		

DINNER								
	Dinner Totals							
	Blood Glucose Level	Befor:				Time:		
		After:				Time:		

SNACKS								
	Snack Totals							

Daily Totals							

Bedtime Blood Glucose Level		Time:	

Water	Sleep	Medication	Activity	Minutes	Notes

Diabetes Log Book

Date:						M	T	W	T	F	S	S

	Meal	Cal	Fat	Carbs	Total Sugar	Added Sugar	Protein	Fiber
BREAKFAST								
	Breakfast Totals							
	Blood Glucose Level	Befor:			Time:			
		After:			Time:			
LUNCH								
	Lunch Totals							
	Blood Glucose Level	Befor:			Time:			
		After:			Time:			
DINNER								
	DinnerTotals							
	Blood Glucose Level	Befor:			Time:			
		After:			Time:			
SNACKS								
	Snack Totals							

Daily Totals						

Bedtime Blood Glucose Level		Time:	

Water	Sleep	Medication	Activity	Minutes	Notes

Diabetes Log Book

Date:						M	T	W	T	F	S	S

	Meal	Cal	Fat	Carbs	Total Sugar	Added Sugar	Protein	Fiber
BREAKFAST								
	Breakfast Totals							
	Blood Glucose Level	Befor:				Time:		
		After:				Time:		

LUNCH								
	Lunch Totals							
	Blood Glucose Level	Befor:				Time:		
		After:				Time:		

DINNER								
	Dinner Totals							
	Blood Glucose Level	Befor:				Time:		
		After:				Time:		

SNACKS								
	Snack Totals							

Daily Totals							

Bedtime Blood Glucose Level		Time:	

Water	Sleep	Medication	Activity	Minutes	Notes

Diabetes Log Book

Date:				M T W T F S S			

	Meal	Cal	Fat	Carbs	Total Sugar	Added Sugar	Protein	Fiber
BREAKFAST								
	Breakfast Totals							
	Blood Glucose Level	Befor:			Time:			
		After:			Time:			
LUNCH								
	Lunch Totals							
	Blood Glucose Level	Befor:			Time:			
		After:			Time:			
DINNER								
	Dinner Totals							
	Blood Glucose Level	Befor:			Time:			
		After:			Time:			
SNACKS								
	Snack Totals							

Daily Totals							

Bedtime Blood Glucose Level		Time:	

Water	Sleep	Medication	Activity	Minutes	Notes

Diabetes Log Book

Date:					M	T	W	T	F	S	S

	Meal	Cal	Fat	Carbs	Total Sugar	Added Sugar	Protein	Fiber
BREAKFAST								
	Breakfast Totals							
	Blood Glucose Level	Befor:				Time:		
		After:				Time:		
LUNCH								
	Lunch Totals							
	Blood Glucose Level	Befor:				Time:		
		After:				Time:		
DINNER								
	Dinner Totals							
	Blood Glucose Level	Befor:				Time:		
		After:				Time:		
SNACKS								
	Snack Totals							

Daily Totals							

Bedtime Blood Glucose Level		Time:	

Water	Sleep	Medication	Activity	Minutes	Notes

Notes

Diabetes Log Book

| Date: | | | | | | M T W T F S S | | | |

	Meal	Cal	Fat	Carbs	Total Sugar	Added Sugar	Protein	Fiber
BREAKFAST								
	Breakfast Totals							
	Blood Glucose Level	Befor:			Time:			
		After:			Time:			

LUNCH								
	Lunch Totals							
	Blood Glucose Level	Befor:			Time:			
		After:			Time:			

DINNER								
	Dinner Totals							
	Blood Glucose Level	Befor:			Time:			
		After:			Time:			

SNACKS								
	Snack Totals							

Daily Totals							

Bedtime Blood Glucose Level		Time:	

Water	Sleep	Medication	Activity	Minutes	Notes

Diabetes Log Book

Date:					M T W T F S S			

	Meal	Cal	Fat	Carbs	Total Sugar	Added Sugar	Protein	Fiber
BREAKFAST								
	Breakfast Totals							
	Blood Glucose Level	Befor:				Time:		
		After:				Time:		

LUNCH								
	Lunch Totals							
	Blood Glucose Level	Befor:				Time:		
		After:				Time:		

DINNER								
	Dinner Totals							
	Blood Glucose Level	Befor:				Time:		
		After:				Time:		

SNACKS								
	Snack Totals							

Daily Totals							

Bedtime Blood Glucose Level		Time:	

Water	Sleep	Medication	Activity	Minutes	Notes

Diabetes Log Book

Date:					M T W T F S S			

	Meal	Cal	Fat	Carbs	Total Sugar	Added Sugar	Protein	Fiber
BREAKFAST								
	Breakfast Totals							
	Blood Glucose Level	Befor:				Time:		
		After:				Time:		

		Cal	Fat	Carbs	Total Sugar	Added Sugar	Protein	Fiber
LUNCH								
	Lunch Totals							
	Blood Glucose Level	Befor:				Time:		
		After:				Time:		

		Cal	Fat	Carbs	Total Sugar	Added Sugar	Protein	Fiber
DINNER								
	Dinner Totals							
	Blood Glucose Level	Befor:				Time:		
		After:				Time:		

SNACKS								
	Snack Totals							

Daily Totals							

Bedtime Blood Glucose Level		Time:	

Water	Sleep	Medication	Activity	Minutes	Notes

Diabetes Log Book

| Date: | | | | | M T W T F S S | | | |

	Meal	Cal	Fat	Carbs	Total Sugar	Added Sugar	Protein	Fiber
BREAKFAST								
	Breakfast Totals							
	Blood Glucose Level	Befor:				Time:		
		After:				Time:		

LUNCH								
	Lunch Totals							
	Blood Glucose Level	Befor:				Time:		
		After:				Time:		

DINNER								
	Dinner Totals							
	Blood Glucose Level	Befor:				Time:		
		After:				Time:		

SNACKS								
	Snack Totals							

Daily Totals								

Bedtime Blood Glucose Level		Time:	

Water	Sleep	Medication	Activity	Minutes	Notes

Notes

Thank you!

WE ARE GLAD THAT YOU PURCHASED OUR BOOK!
PLEASE LET US KNOW HOW WE CAN IMPROVE IT!
YOUR FEEDBACK IS ESSENTIAL TO US.

Contact us at:

M log'Sin@gmail.com

JUST TITLE THE EMAIL 'CREATIVE' AND WE WILL

GIVE YOU SOME EXTRA SURPRISES!

www.ingramcontent.com/pod-product-compliance
Lightning Source LLC
Chambersburg PA
CBHW071435210326
41597CB00020B/3808